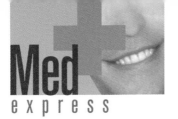

Med
express

overcoming
headaches

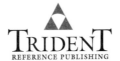

TRIDENT
REFERENCE PUBLISHING

Published by:
Trident Reference Publishing
801 12th Avenue South, Suite 400
Naples, Fl 34102 USA
Phone: + 1 239 649 7077
Email: sales@trident-international.com
Website: www.trident-international.com

Overcoming Headaches
© Trident Reference Publishing

Publisher
Simon St. John Bailey

Editor-in-chief
Isabel Toyos

Art Director
Aline Talavera

Photos
© Trident Reference Publishing, © Getty Images,
© Jupiter Images, © Planstock, © J. Alonso

Includes index
ISBN 1582799636 (hc)
UPC 615269996362 (hc)
ISBN 1582799512 (pbk)
UPC 615269995129 (pbk)

2005 Edition
Printed in USA

overcoming headaches

 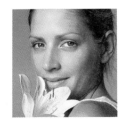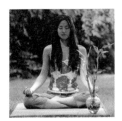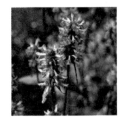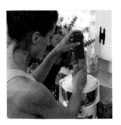

What are headaches?

At least 50 percent of people has suffered from headaches at some point in their lives. Headaches are a common ailment that can arise from a number of physical problems. There are also different types of headaches; some of them transitory and others chronic, which require specific treatment.

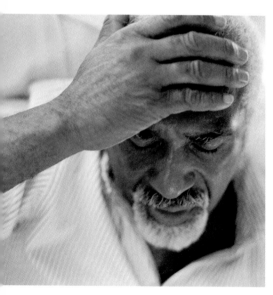

✚ The classic headache is mostly related to a number of common ailments such as digestive problems (excessive foods, indulgence in alcohol, gastrointestinal disorders, indigestion caused by greasy foods, constipation), altered vision, sinus infections, muscle contractions and tension. This type of headache is more or less easy to treat. Very different are migraines, which tend to be recurring and chronic. Migraine pain is moderate to severe, often described as pounding, throbbing pain in the skull. The exact causes of migraines are unknown, although they may be diagnosed by previous symptoms such as disturbances of vision and/or nausea. Among those symptoms is the sense of seeing "little lights", light sensitivity (staying away from lighted places because bright lights are bothersome) and other ailments that accompany the pain such as irritability, vomiting and loss of appetite.

Migraine headaches tend to run in families, but the exact mechanism of inheritance is not understood. The causes of migraines are related to blood vessel contractions, other changes in the brain and other inherited abnormalities such as hormonal problems. Recurring migraines should be treated by a doctor and require special medical attention. Headaches can also be caused by high blood pressure, generally occuring in the back of the neck, at the base of the skull, these require immediate medical attention.

URBAN ENVIRONMENT HEADACHES
Tension headaches are considered an environmental ailment because outside factors tend to be the most frequent cause such as bad body posture, stress, depression and a fast paced lifestyle.

TYPES OF HEADACHES

Migraines. Intense pain on one side of the head always repeated in the same area. It is accompanied by disturbances of vision and hearing, nausea and vomiting.

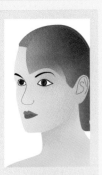

Headaches caused by digestive problems. Headaches accompanied by stomach, kidney, intestinal and gallbladder ailments. Sometimes linked with overindulgence of alcohol, food sensitivities and food additives.

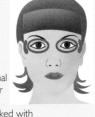

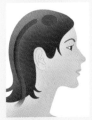

Stress headaches. Pain runs from the neck to the top of the skull.

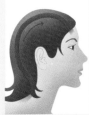

Tension headaches. These muscle contraction headaches cause mild to moderate pain from the neck to the forehead.

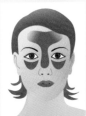

Sinus headaches. Inflammation of the lining of one of the eight sinus cavities can cause a deep, dull, chronic ache around the eyes, nose and head.

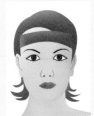

Anxiety headaches. Pain crosses the forehead.

How to treat headaches

The vast majority of headaches are harmless and can be treated with a pain reliever. However, self-treating headaches may run risks and rather than treating the problem you may just be getting accustomed to medicines. There are a number of natural remedies that may be effective in treating and preventing headaches.

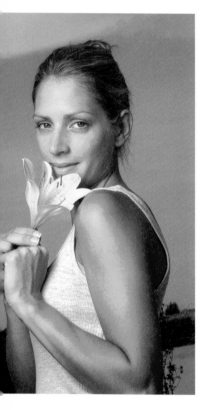

When you suffer from recurring headaches, it's important to analyze the situations where they occur. This will help you to identify what triggers your symptoms: foods, excessive smoking or alcohol, lack of exercise, environmental factors or taking new medication. This way you will be able to begin to control the ailment. When you experience occasional pain that tends to go away after a few hours. Resting in a calm dark room, taking a hot shower or receiving a comforting massage with essential oils may relieve your symptoms. However, if your pain is persistent or recurring you should see a doctor.

MEDICAL TREATMENT

It is never good to self-treat your symptoms, even if your headaches are harmless, because if you take over the counter painkillers longer than advised by pharmaceutical companies and avoid going to the doctor, your headaches may rebound. That's to say that they will reappear and may worsen if you don't treat them with

COMPLEMENTARY REMEDIES

Holistic treatment may be very useful in treating tension headaches or headaches brought on by unhealthy lifestyle habits. This can help you to harmonize and release daily tensions, which may help to prevent headaches and treat recurring headaches. The most recommended include:

- *Herbal remedies in infusions and decoctions.*
- *Aromatherapy (essential oils and compresses).*
- *Yoga.*
- *Shiatsu.*
- *Chinese massages*
- *and do-it-yourself massages.*
- *Reflexology.*
- *Hydrotherapy.*
- *Diet for specific needs (low-fat foods that maintain constant blood sugar level, see* Healing foods *on page 46).*

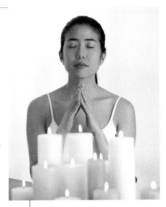

pain relieving medication. This causes a vicious cycle of taking medication not to treat or fight the ailment, but to prevent the pain from reappearing. Chronically taking painkillers like aspirin can bring on side effects; for example blood clotting, traumas to the digestive track such as ulcers and other physical changes.

There are a number of natural complementary remedies that might help to relieve symptoms. Holistic treatments such as tinctures and exercise can play an important role in treating headaches, sometimes providing immediate relief without side effects or creating dependency.

IMMEDIATE TREATMENT

Here are some simple strategies for relieving headaches:

- Lying down in a silent, dark room. Close the curtains, turn off the TV and disconnect the telephone. Next, relax your jaw as much as you can. Inhale and exhale deeply while you relax your muscles, one by one. It is positive to visualize beautiful scenery or landscapes, or to imagine a silent place to take you away and help you mentally and physically relax.
- Take a hot shower and let the water hit your tense muscles that tend to trigger headaches.
- Have someone massage your temples or neck, or use do-it-yourself massage techniques.

Healthy lifestyle

Keeping a healthy lifestyle, good diet and exercising regularly can help to fight stress and the many factors that cause anxiety, which may prevent headaches.

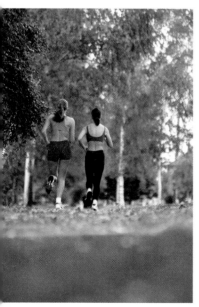

✚ The likelihood of suffering from a headache reduces when you learn to manage stressful situations and psychological and emotional tensions and maintain a healthy rhythm. With the help of a specialist you can identify what daily lifestyle habits may contribute to recurring headaches. Some general recommendations include:

◼ **Sleeping well**

You should try to keep a regular sleeping schedule, maintaining a set time for going to bed and waking up, making sure to get a minimum amount of 7 hours sleep a night. Next, try to adjust the rest of your daily activities to a strict schedule. The body needs repairing sleep, which is fundamental to prevent insomnia and restoring rest. Using a comfortable mattress, avoiding eating right before going to bed and avoiding excess coffee, alcohol and cigarettes may help you to sleep better.

◼ **Eating healthy food**

Eating a healthy diet isn't limited to only avoiding certain foods and eating others (see *Headache fighting foods*, on page 46), but is important to keep a regular schedule to eat without being in a hurry. In addition, try to follow a balanced diet and eat the four traditional meals: breakfast, lunch, snack and dinner.

■ Regularly exercising

If you haven't kept a regular exercise routine, it's recommended to walk daily, starting with 15 minutes a day and increasing the time as your body feels stronger, until you can walk an hour a day. It is also good to practice sports or to lift weights, which when practiced in moderation can help to prevent bad posture (especially the shoulders and curved back). If you work sitting for long periods of time or work in front of a computer, it's highly recommended to take a few minutes every hour to relieve muscular tension in the shoulder and neck by flexing the muscles in the back (stretching forward and backward), while you raise your chin, close your eyes and breath deeply.

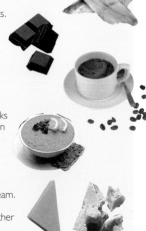

FOODS TO AVOID

- Chocolate.

- Sausages, deli meats, pate and cured meats.

- Canned fish, pickled herring, shellfish and game meat.

- Aged or fermented cheeses.

- Coffee, tea, cola drinks and chocolate milk (in excess).

- Alcoholic drinks (especially beer).

- Butter and whole cream.

- Olives, pickles and other pickled vegetables.

- Lentils, chick peas, cabbage and onion.

■ Reducing stress

Sometimes it's not possible to avoid all types of situations that cause stress, you can try different strategies to reduce daily tension. For example, practicing basic relaxation and meditation techniques may help. You may want to learn different techniques to face difficult situations and whenever necessary, consult a psychotherapist.

Tension fighting yoga

Because tension and anxiety often bring on headaches, different yoga poses —which favor relaxation— may be very beneficial to prevent and relieve headaches and migraines.

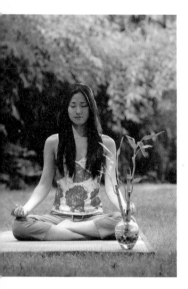

✚ Yoga can be a very beneficial exercise, because the technique guides students to lead a healthy and regular life, which has a lot to do in stress prevention and the accumulation of tension in the body. Through the practice of yoga, energy is channelled constructively, helping us to calm our minds and bringing well-being. This discipline helps oxygen flow to the brain (which helps to reduce irritability) and helps to align the muscles in the head, neck and throughout the entire body. Yoga poses can also help to control the flow of blood to the head and to reduce muscular tension.

Yoga is also highly recommended for patients who can't take medication, because the technique may work as a natural treatment, short term or long term.

THE POSTURES

Each yoga pose (also known as *asanas*) is thought to strengthen, harmonize and increase the body's flexibility. The poses help the mind to concentrate and prepare the body for relaxation through exercises and breathing techniques. It's best to practice yoga sessions in an appropriate atmosphere, with soft lighting, music and repetitive mental formulas (*mantras*) which help you enter a state of meditation. In general, *asanas* help the mind and body to relax, which may be very helpful in preventing and relieving headaches. However, there are a few yoga postures that specifically focus on the energy centers located in the head, that irrigate brain's blood vessels and help fight intense pains.

The Plow

This posture aims to help enter an optimum state of relaxation and mental calm, which may relieve and prevent neurological pain. In addition it nourishes the spinal nerves and gives flexibility to the spine, neck and back, which may help to relieve headaches brought on by tension. This pose also supports digestion, which can sometimes cause headaches.

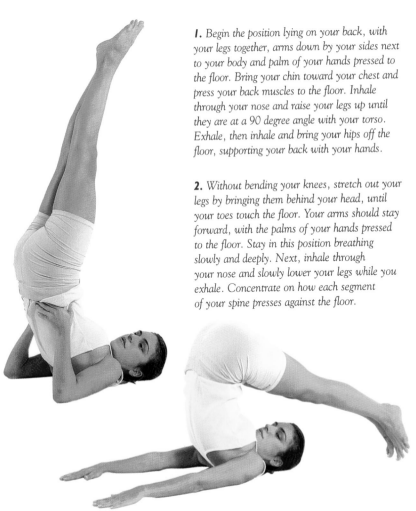

1. Begin the position lying on your back, with your legs together, arms down by your sides next to your body and palm of your hands pressed to the floor. Bring your chin toward your chest and press your back muscles to the floor. Inhale through your nose and raise your legs up until they are at a 90 degree angle with your torso. Exhale, then inhale and bring your hips off the floor, supporting your back with your hands.

2. Without bending your knees, stretch out your legs by bringing them behind your head, until your toes touch the floor. Your arms should stay forward, with the palms of your hands pressed to the floor. Stay in this position breathing slowly and deeply. Next, inhale through your nose and slowly lower your legs while you exhale. Concentrate on how each segment of your spine presses against the floor.

Massaging the pain away

Some relaxing and tension relieving massages may be very effective in relieving headaches.

✚ To help reduce and relieve headaches there are specific massages on the neck, shoulders, shoulder blades, back, temples, forehead, jaw and behind the ears. These massages are relaxing and help to get rid of pain caused by tension in certain parts of the body. You can do these massages yourself, although they are most efficient when done by someone else, especially by a trained massage therapist.

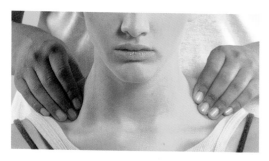

1. In a seated, comfortable position, massage the back of the neck, shoulders and temples.

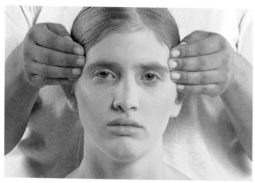

2. First press firmly on the shoulders and then press with your fingertips on the back of the neck and temples (the hands should be lubricated with a neutral oil mixed with three drops of an essential oil —try lavender, camomile or mint).

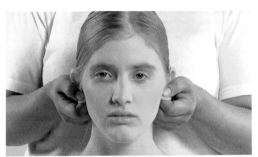

3. With both thumbs, massage the ear lobes. This technique is very important because most nervous tension passes through this part of the body.

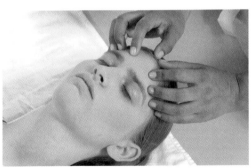

4. With your index and middle fingers, lightly press on the temples. Next, gently massage, using circular movements to relieve pain.

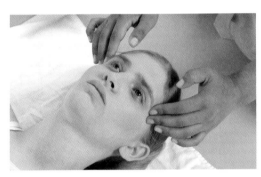

5. Gently press with your fingertips on the middle of the forehead, the area where the ajna or third eye chakra is found. This massage is very efficient for relaxing the mind and getting rid of anxiety.

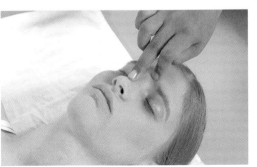

6. Place your fingertips in the area below and above the eyebrows and apply pressure for a few seconds. This pressure helps to relax the mind and to soothe pain, it is ideal for days when you are extremely tired.

Harmonizing shiatsu

Shiatsu is a traditional Oriental technique dating back thousands of years, involving finger pressure. It can fight against headaches, especially those brought on by stress.

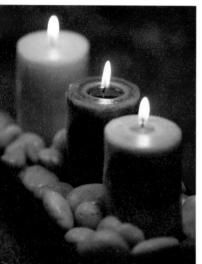

➕ *Shiatsu* is a technique that originated in Oriental medicine, using finger pressure to treat the meridian channels in the body to put our *chi* or life energy into balance. This treatment is recommended for treating stress and can also be beneficial for headaches, neck and shoulder pains.

The technique gathers the excess of energy found in some areas of the body and redistributes this energy where it is most needed, to correct internal imbalances.

In general this massage is practiced on the floor, using a padded exercise or wicker mat. The massage practitioner not only uses the fingers and palms of the hands, but also the elbows, knees and feet to apply pressure to the skin and muscles on key points, to relieve and correct imbalances, eliminate tension and to stimulate the body's ability to self-cure ailments. When a holistic therapist uses *shiatsu*, he treats ailments on a personalized basis. A healthy individual will feel better after a few sessions which serve to relax and regenerate the patient's energy. However, a person highly affected by stress, headaches, stiff neck and back will need at least one weekly session for several months, or more in severe cases. To use simple massages, *shiatsu* can be used at home following the instructions we've put together.

FACE MASSAGES

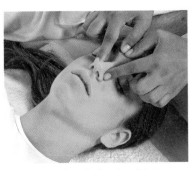

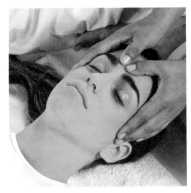

1. Place the thumbs on the forehead and use gentle, yet firm pressure.

3. Massage along both sides of the nose with the index finger and thumb. Next, massage up the bridge of the nose (this point is called the "bright light") and press. This will provide a pleasant effect for tired vision.

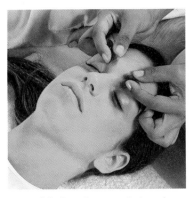

2. Pinch both eyebrows with the index finger and thumb, moving from the center to the temples. Repeat several times to soothe pains in the forehead.

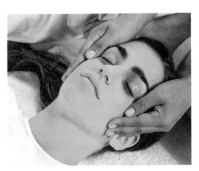

4. Massage along the sides of the face and moving down the cheeks. This is a good technique that may relieve tension stored in the face.

5. Press again on the forehead with the thumbs and rub outward. Next, remain for a few minutes, calm and silent for complete relaxation.

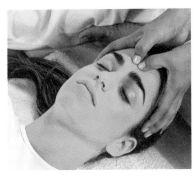

Secret Chinese finger techniques

Among the different manual therapies, Chinese massages may be particularly effective in treating headaches, neck tension and fatigue.

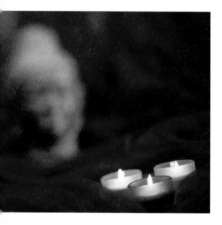

✚ An expert in Chinese massage can work wonders by simply transmitting *chi* (vital energy) to someone who is suffering from headaches. The concept of *chi* is fundamental to life according to Chinese and Japanese traditional medicine. It means vitality, acts as the creating force of the Universe and flows through all living beings. Each human has this energy, although in different levels. Some have weak *chi*, while others have stronger *chi* energy flowing throughout their bodies. Health depends on a strong presence of *chi*, a lack of or imbalances in it can provoke illnesses. Meanwhile, the presence of *chi* helps a person to stay physically and mentally healthy.

Maintaining the life energy balance isn't necessarily easy to achieve, it requires extensive training. However, a trained *chi* can be very efficient in relieving pain. To balance and stimulate life energy flow, the hands are placed on different points of the head. Some massages can be used as self-administered, but most exercises require two people: a donator –sensitive to the process of transmission and receiving– and a receiver.

FOR A COMMON HEADACHE

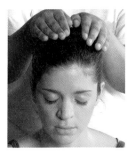

1. The patient should sit in a comfortable position. The person giving the massage places their hands over the head of the receiver, keeping the hands cupped. Concentrate on transmitting chi for two minutes. The receiver should feel a sense of heat in some parts of the head.

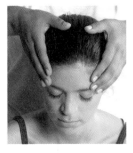

2. Place the index and middle fingers near the eyebrows and transmit the chi to this point for another two minutes. Next, slowly remove the fingers from this point.

FOR MIGRAINES

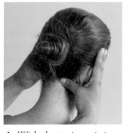

1. With the patient sitting, place the thumbs in the cavities at the base of the skull, right where the neck begins, and transmit chi. One side of the neck may be tenser than the other.

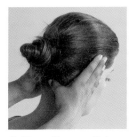

2. Depending on which side is tenser, turn the head toward the right or left until the tension is balanced.

3. Bring the head backward and press with your thumbs the hollows at the base of the skull and transmit chi for a minute.

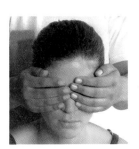

4. Then release the pressure and return the head to its normal position. Place the hands over the eyes and continue transmitting chi for thirty seconds more.

Do-it-yourself massages

These self-massages are ideal for fighting against headaches. They are simple, they don't require too much preparation and can be done at any moment.

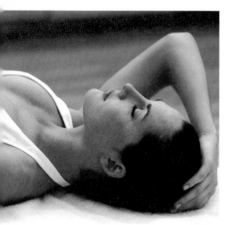

✚ Through massage –an ancient art derived from Oriental philosophy– techniques have been developed over time by a series of cultures, as a form of using the hands to relax, release tension, eliminate toxins, increase muscle tone, relieve pain and to increase the over all health and well-being. Massages are basically sedatives and pleasant therapies.

Some techniques can be applied as self-massages and may be very practical and efficient, especially for intense or chronic headaches. They can be done at any time (any time when you feel achy or you want to relieve tension), although it is recommended to do these self-massages after taking a bath. They can be given directly on the skin's surface, or using a cream or essential oil. It is good to accompany do-it-yourself massages with soft music, to help you to fully relax.

■ **Exercise 1**

To relieve headaches and migraines, press the point on your hand between your index finger and thumb right where the bones meet.

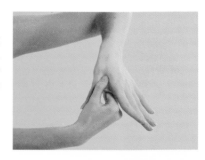

■ Exercise 2

To relieve headaches, especially when they are related to sinus infections, place your thumbs on the edges of where your eyebrows end and stimulate this point by placing the weight of your head on your thumbs.

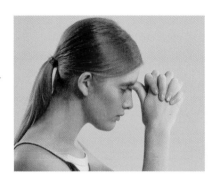

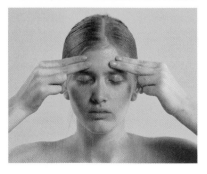

WARNING

These massages present side effects if you have an infection. They should not be used if you have pain caused by an earache or pain in the jaw area, as a result of a tooth infection.

■ Exercise 3

1. To soothe pains in the head, gently press on your temples with the tips of your fingers and use small circular motions (you can alternate between massaging forward and backward).

2. Without stopping, using circular rubbing motions, run your hands along your head, from your temples all the way to the base of your skull and massage this area for a few minutes, also using circular motions.

3. Return to your forehead and massage the area, using circular motions with your index and middle fingers.

Massages area-by-area

There are a number of specific massages that may relieve headaches, depending on the area affected by the pain.

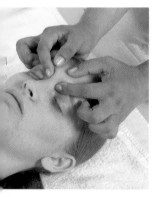

Headaches have different origins and depending on the case can present different characteristics. This is why some headaches are concentrated in the forehead while others are concentrated in the neck, eyes, top of the head or all over the head. There are specific massages for each type of headache, which is why it's good to know what is the cause of the headache. Always accompany complementary therapies with a visit to your doctor.

▲ On the forehead
Stress, digestive changes or sinus infections can cause specific pains in the forehead.
Apply pressure with the tips of your index fingers on each point on the eyebrows and massage using circular motions.

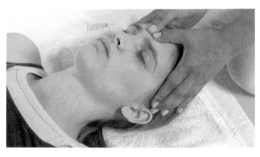

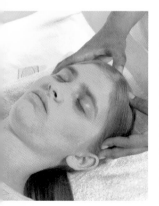

◄ On the eyes and behind the eyes
This is a distinctive pain, which tends to be related to digestive disorders or tired vision.
Press with your index, middle, and ring fingers on the sides of the skull, where the reflex points that correspond to this pain are located.

▲ From the neck to the skull
This intense pain is generally related to stress or problems with posture, especially from stiff necks.
Press with your thumbs on the middle of the forehead, the third eye area. Then smoothe the fingers, massaging in circles, across the forehead to the temples until the nape of the neck at the base of the cranium.

▶ From the nape of the neck to the crown

This can be a very intense pain, generally linked to stress or postural defects, in particular muscle spasms in the neck.

Press the points related to the cervical vertebrae found at the nape of the neck. This is a critical area as it is very vulnerable to tension and bad posture. It is also the point where the nerves meet, radiating pain to the neck, head and shoulders.

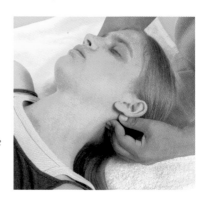

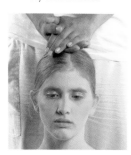

◀ From the neck to the forehead or to the top of the skull

This is an effective technique for all types of headaches related to problems with stress or pains in the base of the skull or neck.

Massage the entire head with the tips of your fingers of both hands, using circular movements, from the skull all the way to the sides of your neck.

▼ All over the head

Pain all over the head tends to be rooted in a series of problems, from a stiff neck and forehead caused by anxiety and tension.

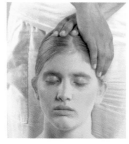

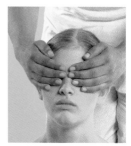

1. *Place the hands above the head. Next, with your palms together, apply gentle taps in a circular motion over the head.*

2. *Place one hand over the head and massage moving from the sides.*

3. *Place the hands over the eyes to complete a relaxation session.*

Relief from the feet

Reflexology has been used as a natural healing art for thousands of years in China, Malaysia and India. The technique helps overall health and relieves aches and pains by the application of pressure on the base of the foot, toes, edges of the heel, palms of the hands and upper part of the hands. Reflexology can be an excellent treatment to relieve headaches.

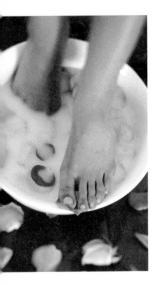

In the early 20th century, US physician William Fitzgerald developed the ancient Oriental healing art of reflexology to relieve pains into a usable diagnostic therapy. Modern reflexology has been pioneered and is widely used in the East and West. Today, this healing art is one of the most extensive alternative therapies in the treatment of common headaches.

The art is based on the principle and study of the reflexes in the body –especially on the hands and feet– that correspond to the body's organs and glands. Applying stimulation and pressure to the feet or hands has similar effects to a total body massage.

In reflexology the body is divided into ten zones, based on a longitudinal guide, from the head to the feet. The right hand and foot corresponds to the right side of the body, while the left hand and foot corresponds to the left side. The base of the foot, the palms of the hand are divided into horizontal zones, which are represented as a mirror image of the entire body.

The area of the toes represents the senses. This is where the nerve endings for the head, eyes, ears, teeth, mouth, throat and neck are found.

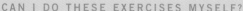

CAN I DO THESE EXERCISES MYSELF?

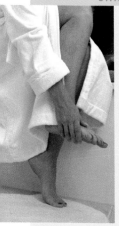

Although it's not the same effect as seeing a practicing reflexologist, you can do some of these reflexology massages yourself for positive effects, especially to relieve intense headaches. Special preparation is not necessary, although it's best to do these massages on bare feet, so that you can reach the reflex points more exactly. You should sit in a comfortable position –a position in which you don't have to bend your back too much–, if possible with your knee bent, legs crossed and one of your feet placed on your thigh, so that you can have a better visual perspective of your foot. Over time you may develop further sensitivity with your fingers and so won't have to use your eyes as your guide. You can follow, when first beginning these massages, a fixed routine, paying special attention to the points which are giving you problems (see diagram).

For headaches you should concentrate and apply pressure on the big toe, all the points that correspond to the head are on this toe, located in the higher area of the toe's tip, near the toenail.

Each one represents that when pressure is applied to these reflex points on the toes, the pressure affects the entire area of the head, brain and senses. As a method of diagnosis and treatment, reflexology may be very effective in relieving pain. Reflexology is a pleasant treatment that acts as a healthy, relaxing, and non-invasive therapy, which stimulates the body's ability to cure itself.

POINTS THAT REFLECT THE HEAD

The feet reflects the entire body; this is why when pressing on a certain area of the foot you are in essence working that part of the body. There are specific points located on the toes that correspond to the sinuses, brain, eyes, ears, throat and neck.

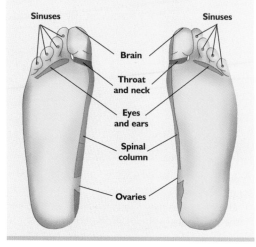

Sinuses
Sinuses
Brain
Throat and neck
Eyes and ears
Spinal column
Ovaries

EXERCISES AGAINST PAIN

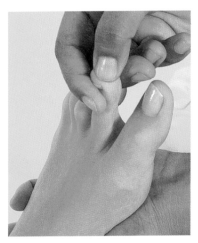

1. Apply pressure with the thumb on all of the tips of the toes to release energy.

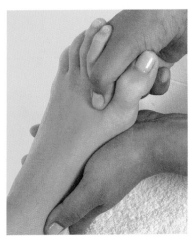

2. Press on the point located between the big toe and second toe. This will help to relieve headaches caused by states of nervousness.

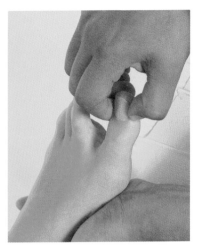

3. Apply pressure on both sides of the big toe, right in the hollow area where the toenail begins. This movement is indicated for headaches caused by an inflamed liver.

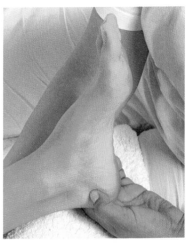

4. When ovary problems or premenstrual tension causes your headaches, press on the areas that reflect those areas located on the heel.

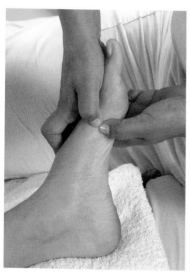

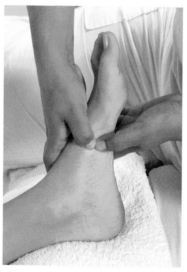

5. *To relieve headaches caused by congestion in the spinal column, apply pressure with the thumb on the place that corresponds to this point, located on the inner edge of the foot.*

6. *To treat the spinal disk, which when swollen can cause headaches, press on the point that corresponds to the spinal column, in the center of the inner edge of the foot.*

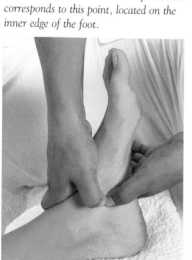

7. *To treat swollen muscles in the back, apply pressure on the inner edge of the foot, where the heel begins.*

HERBS AND ESSENTIAL OILS

To increase the therapeutic effects of healing baths, you can add fresh herbs or a few drops of essential oils to the water. The most common essential oils made from a base of herbs include camomile, ginger, sage, cedar wood, lemon, rose and tea tree oil (see Essential oils from A to Z, on page 31).

Serenity with water

For thousands of years ancient cultures have used water as a natural medicine to treat a number of ailments, especially those brought on by stress or excessive tension. It is an effective therapy for many ailments, including headaches.

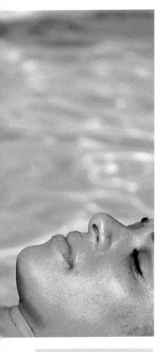

Egyptians, Chinese, Hebrews, Greeks and native Americans used sources of water for their healing properties to treat illnesses and injuries. Today, the method of using water therapeutically has been readopted and introduced as a beauty treatment, to relieve inflammations, to relax muscles and for its detoxifying and purifying properties. In addition hydrotherapy may work wonders against stress, which is why this therapy is so commonly used to treat symptoms related to backaches, anxiety and headaches.

WASHING THE FEET AND HANDS

Footbaths may be a very beneficial therapy for relieving headaches, but you should take certain precautions such as using this remedy in a warm room to avoid colds and flu. It's most effective to use this therapy before going to bed, cover up well directly after the bath. Soak your feet, covering the entire foot up to the ankles, with hot water for 15 minutes. Simultaneously apply a cold compress on your head. The hot water will stimulate and open the blood vessels in your feet and the cold compress will constrict the blood vessels in the brain, which may help the pain to disappear. For the foot bath you can alternate hot and cold water. You may use the therapy that

NOTE
You should always consult your physician before taking hydrotherapy practices.

stimulates and affects the points on the feet that reflect the nerves.

COMPRESSES

For headaches, compresses may be the most effective therapy to relieve pain. Use linen clothes soaked in cold water. Wring the cloth out and fold several times. Apply to the head for 10 minutes.

SOAKING BATHS

Baths are great to relax you, reduce your anxiety and to relieve chronic pain; they are used to stimulate and improve blood circulation. It's best to take warm baths when the water temperature is between 97 to 100°F/36 to 38°C and to stay in the water for 20 minutes. After taking a bath, dry off and cover up, cozy in bed and rest for 30 to 40 minutes.

STEAM

As steam decongests, it may be used to relieve headaches caused by colds and flu. Breath steam from boiling water (you can use water alone or with aromatic herbs) for 10 to 15 minutes. Afterward, cover up or lie down in bed for at least half an hour, until you stop sweating. If you add herbs to the water, it's best to use those recommended for headaches (see *Essential oils from A to Z*, on page 31).

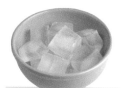

APPLYING ICE
You can use this therapy as a pain reliever and to reduce swelling. Wrap crushed ice in a towel, cover with plastic and apply to the head, in the spot where you are experiencing pain. You should keep the ice pack on the area for no more than 10 minutes; take a break and repeat if necessary.

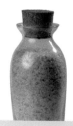

HOME SPA

When your headaches are caused by excess tension, a spa –which can be found in almost any city or town– can be a great way to relieve your pain. However, you can also create a temporary spa in your home, using different therapies to relax, increase your physical health and to relieve pain: using soaking baths with essential aromatic oils, massaging shower heads, steam baths, saunas and Jacuzzi. These are great sedative techniques to relax your muscles and to relieve the tensions built up from straining daily activities.

More solutions

Acupuncture, gem therapy, chromotherapy, and magnetic therapy
may work as other effective alternative remedies for headaches.
We've put together a brief summary of each.

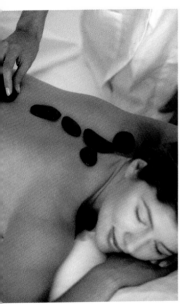

These "energy therapies" or "vibration therapies" work on the body's energy centers or central *chi* flows. They may help to prevent and fight against headaches.

ACUPUNCTURE

Acupuncture is an Asian healing technique dating back thousands of years and has been accepted by modern medicine as a complementary therapy. According to the theory of acupuncture, pain blocks the flow of vital energy (*chi*). Acupuncture uses the insertion of tiny stainless steal needles to stimulate acupuncture points –located along 12 meridians or energy channels that divide the body– to redirect the *chi*. Many scientific and medical studies have proven that acupuncture can be effective, especially to relieve chronic headaches. Acupuncture is always used as a complementary therapy, accompanied by medical treatment. It not only reduces pain but also improves health, making it possible for the patient to take less medication. This therapy has an immediate sedative and relaxing effect, which makes it a good therapy for sharp, intense pains. It has been discovered that stimulating the nervous system with acupuncture needles releases endorphins –along with other substances– that act as potent pain relievers. You should always see a licensed practitioner.

CHROMOTHERAPY

Chromotherapy, also called color therapy, is the use of the curative powers of color and light. Chromotherapy considers that within our body, our organs, muscles, cells and nerves all have a level of vibration. When our body becomes out of balance, disease occurs. Each color has its own frequency and vibration. Color and light may help bring our physical and emotional systems into balance. Colored light is used as "chromotherapy medicine" (water, oil or sugar energized with color).

Green is calming and sedative, helping to relieve headaches and other similar pains. For fever, headaches and toothaches it's recommended to use blue for its antiseptic and refreshing character. Resting in rooms with this color or going for a stroll in a landscape surrounded by green and blue colors may help to relieve symptoms.

MAGNETIC THERAPY

This alternative treatment uses magnetic fields (biomagnetics or electrobiomagnetics) to treat various physical and emotional conditions. More and more this therapy is used to treat headaches and backaches. The magnets are attached by tape or velcro to certain pain points, for example the base of the skull. The magnet is left on that spot over night or when you take time to relax.

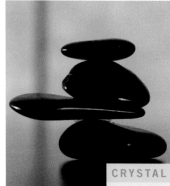

CRYSTAL THERAPY

Crystal therapy dates back to Inca, Egyptian, Mayan, Atlantean, and Lemurian civilizations. Developed by the Veda Hindus, this therapy uses crystals and gem stones to draw and amplify light and color to the body's aura, thus raising its vibrational frequency, and facilitating healing. In this healing practice, quartz, and other stones and crystals are placed on and around the body to stimulate and sensitize subtle vibration patterns, release energy blockages, and harmonize vibration frequencies. They are placed in a special place (for example under your pillow). Amethyst is considered one of the most important gems to cure and very effective against nervous and mental ailments, headaches and stress. For migraines and stiff muscles jade is recommended.

Nature's way of helping

Nature provides us with a number of medicinal plants that can be very helpful in treating our health and fighting against headaches. There are also a number of essential oils (mentioned in the *Essential oils from A to Z* box) for external use, they are extracted from botanical plants and can be used on the skin or for their aroma.

➕ Headaches are generally caused by previous physical problems like high blood pressure, back tension, stress, nervous exhaustion, digestive ailments, tooth aches, visual fatigue, exposure to the sun, sinus infections, etc. The first step in treating headaches is to visit your doctor for an exact medical diagnosis and to treat the cause of the ailment. Essential oils –made from a base of herbs– can act in the form of aromatherapy as an extenuating therapy for migraines and headaches. The following plants are natural remedies that might be considered "headache" herbs. Some herbs may be more difficult to find than others, but there are a number of health food stores that may carry these remedies. In general, they are used fresh or dried or in the form of tinctures, powder and capsules.

> **NOTE**
> You should always consult your physician before starting any herbal treatment.

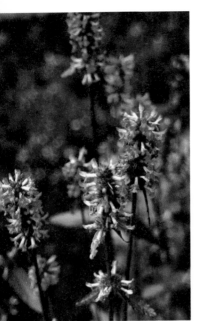

Betony
(*Betonica officinalis*)
• **Parts used.** Flowers and leaves are cultivated during the end of spring until summer. They are dried in a ventilated structure and used in infusions. After the plant is dried, it gives an aromatic smell. It has a bitter

taste. Betony can also be found in powder form.

• It is native to Western and Northern Europe.

• The plant is composed of tannins, alkaloids and glycosides; it is particularly rich in phenolic acids, such as ferulic, chlorogenic and valerianic acids. Glycosides found in plants contribute to their blood pressure controlling properties.

• Betony is recommended for people who suffer from headaches brought on by high blood pressure. It can be used for all headache types for its soothing properties.

• **Warning.** It is important to use precaution with this herb because it can cause vomiting.

Cloves
(Eugenia caryphyllata)

• **Parts used.** The flower buds, which look like nails. The flowers grow on an evergreen tree, native to the Spice Islands and the Philippines but also grown in India, Sumatra, Jamaica, the West Indies and Brazil. In China, during the Han dynasty those who addressed the emperor were required to hold cloves in their mouths to mask bad breath. In China and India it was also used to rub on the gums to sooth toothaches.

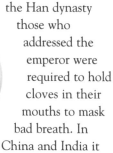

The aroma that fills the dentist's office is a derivative of an essential oil extracted from cloves, used as a natural antiseptic.

AROMATHERAPY

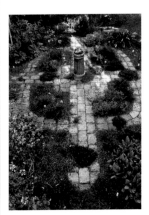

Ancient cultures have long used essential oils derived from plants for their therapeutic properties. The aromas help to energize you, contribute to sedation of attacks, stimulate the senses, calm anger and help to overcome fears or indecision. When you are stiff, with achy and tense muscles throughout the body, taking a bath with essential oils or using them during a massage can work miracles for the body. There are a number of essential oils that have properties that may be useful specifically against headaches. They can be added in massages to help clear the mind, to vapors, cold compresses to apply to the neck or tense shoulders, or to sedative blends perfect for adding to a warm soaking bath. Essential oils should be used under the supervision of a medical professional. In the following pages, we have developed a guide to the most efficient essential oils from A to Z that may work as remedies for headaches.

CALMING CLOVES
To help relieve headaches, nothing is better than an infusion prepared with 3 cloves and 1 cup of boiling water. Allow to steep, cool slightly and drink.

• Cloves can be used to make infusions for rubbings, washing or gargles, used as essential oils, capsules, tinctures or added to ointments.
• Cloves carry potent antibacterial, anti-inflammatory, and pain relieving actions. They also work to prevent scarring. They are especially effective in relieving headaches brought on by toothaches and dental problems.
• **Warning.** It's not recommended for patients who suffer from gastritis, gastric-duodenal ulcers, irritable bowel syndrome, colitis ulcers and some neurological illnesses.

Dandelion
(*Taraxacum officinale*)

• **Parts used.** The leaves and roots, which are prepared in infusions and decoctions.
• Native to Europe and Asia, today it is

cultivated throughout the world. The scientific name comes from the Greek word *taraxos* (disorder) and *aka* (remedy). The plant's flowers are bright yellow, and grow wild around the borders of cultivated land.

• The leaves are a rich source of potassium, which is interesting since the leaves are used for their diuretic action. Because of the leaves' diuretic and detoxifying action they are recommended for excess tension that may provoke headaches and other ailments. In China, dandelion root was used to treat liver, gallbladder, kidney, and joint problems. In some countries, dandelion is considered a blood purifier and used to treat water retention, and diseases of the liver. Because it may help to purify the liver, it may help to relieve headaches caused by excessive rich foods or alcohol.

• **Warning.** In cases of stomach ulcer or gastritis, dandelion should be used cautiously, as it may cause overproduction of stomach acid. In this case dandelion should be used after meals. Over dosage of dandelion can bring on slight diarrhea.

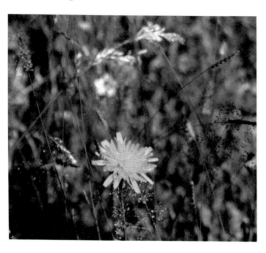

ESSENTIAL OILS
FROM A TO Z

BERGAMOT

This oil, with its fresh, citric, almost floral aroma, is good for headaches caused by stress and mental fatigue. It may also help for cases of depression. It is used in massages and baths.

Safety. This oil increases the skin's sensitivity to sunlight, which you should avoid after using it.

CINNAMON

Warm, sweet, spicy and inviting aroma. This oil may be used against headaches.

Safety. You should always buy essential oil made from cinnamon tree's leaves, because if made from the bark it can irritate the skin. The oil made from the tree's leaves is so potent that it should be used in low doses.

Mad-dog skullcap
(Scutellaria lateriflora)

• **Parts used.** The entire plant is used to prepare infusions or to make tinctures.

• It is also known as the Virginian skullcap, because it grows abundantly in Virginia, USA. The Cherokee Indians used this plant to relieve headaches brought on by premenstrual discomforts.

• Its active components (scutellarin, a flavonoid glycoside and many other flavones) act on the nervous system.

• Has sedative and calming properties, which may be effective for headaches brought on by tension. In general this plant may help to treat and fortify an over-stimulated nervous system. This plant is highly recommended for migraines, alone or combined with other plants such as lavender and passion flower.

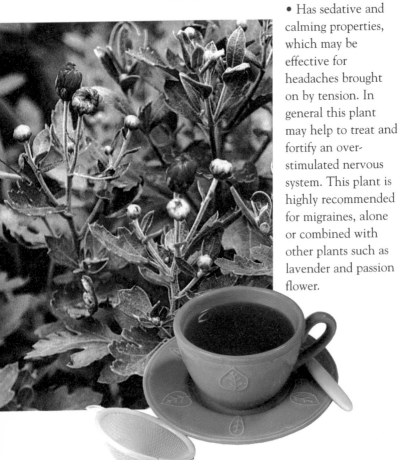

CALMING DROPS OF LAVENDER

For headaches, take 1 1/2 teaspoons of lavender tincture diluted in a glass of water before going to bed. You can also add a few cups of lavender infusion or essential oil to a bathtub before going to bed to relieve stress and tension.

ESSENTIAL OILS FROM A TO Z

FENNEL
Fresh, green and herbal aroma. This essential oil might help to counteract headaches caused by colds and flu. Blends well with thyme.
Safety. Should not be used on pregnant women, children and people who suffer from epilepsy.

GERANIUM
This oil has a floral, earthy, sweet, soft and dry aroma. It may work as an efficient remedy against the anxiety that accompanies headaches. Blends well with rose, sandalwood, sweet marjoram and lavender.
Safety. Shouldn't be used during pregnancy.

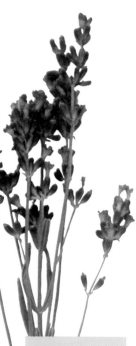

Lavender
(Lavandula officinalis)
• **Parts used.** Flowers and leaves to prepare in infusions or to make essential oils and tinctures.
• The ancient Romans used lavender to perfume water. This plant was introduced to England around 1560 and was taken to the Americas by the first colonists.
• It grows wild in its native Mediterranean, and was used by ancient cultures to fight headaches and exhaustion. In addition, it leaves a lovely, floral scent.
• Today, lavender is used against headaches, depression and insomnia. This plant has calming and relaxing properties.

AROMATIC AND BENEFICIAL TEA
To help fight headaches, prepare an infusion with 1 teaspoon of dried lavender added to 1 cup of boiling water. Allow to steep for 5 minutes, drain and drink.

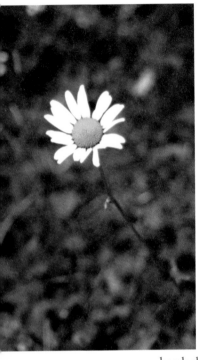

Roman camomile
(*Chamaemelum nobile*)

• **Parts used.** The flowers are used to make infusions.

• It is popularly known as "garden camomile." Also called camomile, derived from the Greek word *kamai* (in the earth) and *melon* (apple).

• Camomile was one of the first herbs taken by European colonists to the New World. In the middle of the XVII century, by religious order in Quebec, it was used as an herbal medicine for various ailments.

• The active ingredients chamazulene, alpha-bisabolol, alpha-bisabolol oxides A & B, apigenin, luteolin, and quercetin have relaxing properties for the nervous system.

• Recommended for fighting headaches and can be used for colds and respiratory problems.

Camomile
(*Chamomilla recutita*)

• **Parts used.** The flowers are used in infusions and also used to make essential oils.

• Also known as "German camomile" or "wild

YELLOW INFUSION

For a remedy that may help to relieve headache add hot water at boiling point to Roman camomile flowers in a bowl. Make sure to cover the preparation so that it doesn't lose the curing properties in the steam. This infusion can be added to baths, to relax adults and little ones.

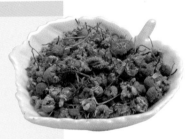

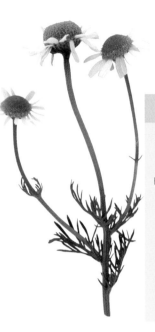

RELAXING CAMOMILE

This infusion of German camomile may help to relieve stress and headaches brought on by certain nervous disorders. Place a generous amount of flowers in a cup and add hot water at boiling point. It's recommended drinking 2 tablespoons 3 time per day.

GINGER

Warm and spicy aroma. This oil is known for its beneficial effects in soothing migraines and nausea caused by motion sickness and other digestive disorders.

Safety. Ginger tends to increase the body's temperature, and can cause discomfort to women who are suffering from hot flashes during menopause.

JUNIPER

Fresh, clean perfume, with a touch of wood. Juniper is a cleansing, purifying and detoxifying oil. Ideal for treating headaches caused by stressful situations, poor diet or excessive use of alcohol.

Safety. Juniper should not be used on pregnant women.

camomile", has more potent properties than Roman camomile or garden camomile.

• This plant has a less bitter flavor than the Roman species. Both varieties grow abundantly in Europe.

• It is recommended, along with ginger, for migraines and motion sickness caused by traveling. Because of its sedative virtues, it helps to relieve stress. Its antispasmodic properties relieve headaches caused by excess tension. It is also recommended for problems related to tired vision.

FENNEL AROMATHERAPY

Essential oil of fennel can be used in massages and compresses to help relieve headaches caused by colds and flu. Mix 1 teaspoon of essential oil to 1 tablespoon with a neutral oil and apply to the temples and between the eyebrows.

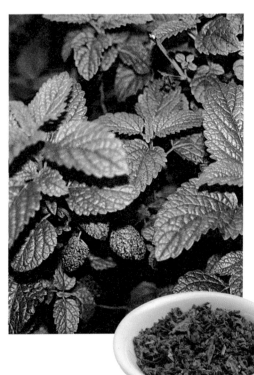

Lemon balm
(Melissa officinalis)

• **Parts used.** The leaves and flowers are used dried or fresh to prepare infusions.

• The scientific name in Greek, means "bee", making reference to the attraction this insect has to this plant.

• Native to Southern Europe, Western Asia and North Africa, although today it is grown throughout the world.

• This plant's properties tend to have relaxing effects and to act on the nervous system. Studies have shown that lemon balm leaves carry properties that calm the central nervous system and soothe headaches brought on by tension. Currently, it is used against anxiety, slight depression and irritability.

• **Warning.** Lemon balm may inhibit the function of the thyroid gland, and presents side effects for patients suffering from underactive thyroid glands. People with normal thyroid gland function, can take lemon balm without any side effects.

HOT TEA TO CLEAR THE MIND

Boil lemon balm flowers in water for 5 minutes, strain and allow to steep. Mix with honey and drink up to 3 cups daily. After 2 or 3 days you might notice positive results.

Pick fresh mint and wash the leaves thoroughly with cold water. Mix with fresh sliced tomatoes and dress with olive oil, apple cider vinegar and sea salt.

Mint
(Menthax piperita)

• **Parts used.** The leaves are used to prepare infusions and to make essential oils.

• The ancient Egyptians used mint for a number of medicinal remedies, especially for headaches and stomach aches. In Greece, Hypocrates considered mint a strong aphrodisiac. Plinius applauded this plant for its pain relieving power and recommended using a crown of mint to increase the mind's power.

• Today, this plant is used to treat a number of ailments (headaches, dizziness) caused by excessive food. It is also recommended for recovering strength lost during fatigue and stress. It can be used to clear a clouded mind.

• **Warning.** It is not recommended for gallstones.

BATH WITH ESSENTIAL OIL OF LAVENDER
To help relieve headaches it is recommended to add a few drops of essential oil of lavender to a bowl with water and moisten a washcloth. Apply the compress to the forehead.

ESSENTIAL OILS FROM A TO Z

LAVENDER

This is one of the most versatile essential oils, that has a number of uses. It may be very effective in fighting headaches, relieving tension and bringing on sleep. For its calming and relaxing properties it can be used all over the body and for specific muscular ailments. It can also be used in creams.
Safety. Lavender oil should never be ingested or added to a baby's bath. The baby may drink the water.

HERB LUISA

Has a lemon, lime aroma, which is very relaxing. Adding this essential oil to massages may be an excellent way to tone the nerves and to counteract headaches. It can also be added to a bath, which has a similar tranquilizing effect.

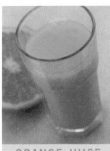

ORANGE JUICE

Juice 2 oranges and add black sugar or honey. Drinking orange juice at breakfast to complement a complete, balanced meal can help to prevent headaches, especially those caused by colds and other respiratory ailments.

Bitter orange
(Citrus aurantium)

• **Parts used.** Fruit and skin.
• In China this fruit is used (ripe or green) for medical treatments, although the un-ripened bitter orange is more potent than the ripe fruit. It is used to balance the nervous system and against insomnia. This fruit's skin is extracted when the fruit is fresh and then dried. In the Middle Ages, this was one of the favorite plants among Arabic doctors.
• Its components –vitamins A, B and C, flavonoids and bitter principles– carry sedative and anti-depressant properties. This fruit also stimulates digestion, and helps to fight against constipation.
• **Warning.** These fruits should be used with caution during pregnancy because they can induce labor contractions.

Rosemary
(Rosmarinus officinalis)

• **Parts used.** The leaves are used in infusions and to make essential oils.
  • Robust perennial, with thin, rigid leaves. Rosemary is considered to be the herb of fidelity.
    • Native to the Mediterranean region, especially central Spain, where it grows in rocky, dry earth.
      • Rosemary's active compounds –rosmarinic acid and other phenolic acids, camphene, camphor, cineole, limonene, linalool,

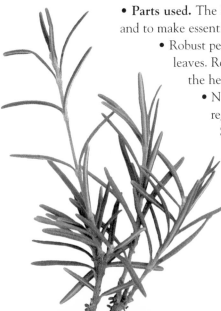

**ROSEMARY FOR
MENTAL FATIGUE**
Cut 1 tomato in halves
and dress with
a pinch of sea salt,
black pepper and plenty
of rosemary ground.

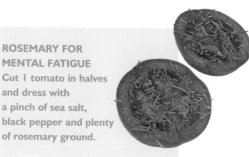

isobutyl acetate, 3-octanone, terpineol, verbenol– are circulatory and nerve stimulants, which in addition to their toning and calming effect on the digestion are used where psychological tension is present. Useful for flatulent dyspepsia, headache or depression associated with debility. Infusions prepared with rosemary leaves have sedative, digestive, anti-oxidant and diuretic properties.

• Externally it may be used to ease muscular pain, sciatica and neuralgia.

• **Warning.** In high doses this plant can be toxic.

MARJORAM
Has an intense herbal aroma, reminiscent of almonds. This oil is a comforting and neural tonic, with pain relieving properties. It may stimulate local blood circulation and is used to treat headaches associated with tension in the neck, with stiff vertebrae. It doesn't present any side effects.

MINT
Refreshing perfume, great for relieving headaches caused by tension. It also helps to clear the head when you need to improve your mental concentration.
Safety. It should not be used by pregnant women or during breastfeeding. It is recommended to use diluted because it can irritate the skin.

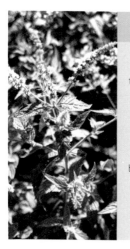

**ESSENTIAL OILS
AGAINST PAIN**

Mint oil is used in many medical clinics in Europe to treat headaches, and has been proven to have positive results. Place 2 to 3 drops of this essential oil over the trigger points (the critical points where headaches begin, generally located on the forehead or frontal sinuses). Massage with the tips of your index and middle fingers for a few minutes in these spots.

White willow
(Salix alba)

• **Parts used.** The leaves, roots and the bark are used and cultivated in the spring. The leaves and roots are used in infusions; the bark should be collected from stems only a few years old, which can only be used in powder form.

• Grows in the wild, along rivers, streams, forests and in other humid environments.

• Among its active components, salicin is the most important for its pain relieving, sedative, anti-rheumatic and anti-fever properties. Hypocrates prescribed remedies of white willow leaves to relieve many problems related to pain. Many ancient cultures used the leaves from this plant, which contain salicylic acid, to treat pain-related ailments.

• White willow can be used as an alternative to an aspirin (acetylsalicylic acid). Many of aspirin's basic components are extracted from this plant, as with ulmaria, before 1890, when aspirin was synthetically produced.

• The dose for average adults is 2 teaspoons dissolved in 1 cup of water once a day.

• **Warning.** People who are allergic to aspirin or other similar medicines should not use white willow. It shouldn't be used on pregnant women or children.

WHITE WILLOW REMEDY FOR HEADACHES

• White willow can be used as an infusion to relieve headaches, using 1 teaspoon of tender leaves in 4 cups of water. It's advised to drink 3 cups a day.

• The leaves can also be used to make a decoction with 2 tablespoons dried white willow bark powder per 4 cups of water. Drink 3 glasses a day, before meals.

• **Warning.** White willow bark has a high concentration of tannins, in some cases 20 percent, which can be harmful to the health if used as a prolonged treatment or in elevated doses.

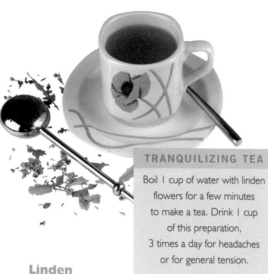

TRANQUILIZING TEA

Boil 1 cup of water with linden
flowers for a few minutes
to make a tea. Drink 1 cup
of this preparation,
3 times a day for headaches
or for general tension.

Linden
(Tilia sp.)

• **Parts used.** The flowers, which properties
are recommended for the nervous system,
particularly for cases of stress or tension.

• In ancient cultures it was said that linden
flowers had a sedative and antispasmodic
effect to treat epilepsy. It was believed that by
placing a patient on a bed of linden flowers,
epileptic attacks would be less serious.

• Native to Europe, today this plant can be
found all around the world.

• It may be very effective for headaches,
especially those caused by colds and
bronchitis. Linden may be beneficial for the
cardiovascular system, moderating blood
pressure. Linden has gained recent fame for
its ability to lower bad cholesterol related
with clogged arteries.

• **Warning.** It is not recommended using
linden if you suffer from high blood pressure.
When taken in high doses it can bring on
insomnia.

NEROLI

This essential oil has a
fresh, pleasant smell
similar to orange
flowers. It is a potent
sedative,
recommended for
cases of stress and
anxiety. Calms the
nerves and helps to
bring on sleep. It may
help to relieve pains
caused by tension,
including headaches.
It doesn't present any
side effects.

OLBAS

This oil, extracted from
olbas, a European herb
whose curative
properties were
discovered in
Switzerland 100 years
ago, is mostly
recommended to treat
headaches.
It stimulates blood
circulation, opens
the pores,
generating warmth and
overall well-being.

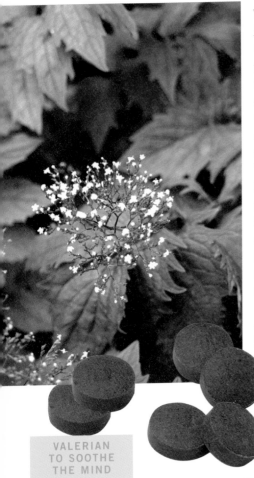

Valerian
(Valeriana officinalis)

• **Parts used.** The roots are prepared in infusions, tinctures, capsules and essential oils.

• Native to Europe and Asia, usually grows on the edges of rivers and streams. Valerian leaves are fernlike. It has tiny flowers -white, pink or lavender- that bloom from late spring through summer. Its scientific name is believed to originate from the Latin word *valere* (health).

• Valerian has a sedative effect, which makes it helpful for fighting headaches. It is recommended for insomnia and for excessive mental activity. It might also work for cases of high blood pressure, when combined with other herbs.

• **Warning.** For some people this herb may have a stimulating effect, rather than a relaxing effect. If this occurs you should immediately stop taking valerian.

VALERIAN TO SOOTHE THE MIND

Take ¹/2 cup of valerian decoction 2 times a day. For headaches and insomnia it's recommended taking I cup during the night. In tincture form, you can take up to 40 drops 3 times a day.

Vervain
(Verbena officinalis)

• **Parts used.** The foliage (fresh and dried) is used to prepare infusions or to make tinctures and capsules.

NATURAL INFUSION

Add hot water (never boiling) to a teapot, along with a handful of fresh vervain leaves. Add honey and allow to sit for 10 minutes. Drink 1 cup regularly, especially after eating a lot. This may be particularly useful for women who suffer from headaches during their menstrual cycle.

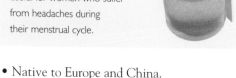

ESSENTIAL OILS FROM A TO Z

SAGE

Its herbal and almond aroma is perfect for relieving chronic headaches caused by excess tension. It helps to clear the mind, though in some people it can produce drowsiness. **Safety.** Shouldn't be used during pregnancy.

SANDALWOOD

Suggestive and spicy perfume, which is helpful in fighting mental and physical exhaustion. It helps cure intense headaches, caused by stress. Favors introspection and meditation.

TEA TREE OIL

Its fresh and slightly spicy aroma, is ideal for relieving dizziness and headaches brought on by colds and flu. **Safety.** It can be used on children over 2 years of age. Should be used in low doses and diluted because it can irritate the skin.

• Native to Europe and China. For centuries it was called the "sacred herb" and "cure-all".

• It is found wild in most of Europe, North Africa and in China and Japan.

• Currently it is used specifically for its re-constructive qualities, to relieve stress and headaches caused by nervous tension. In Chinese medicine vervain is used to treat headaches related to the menstrual cycle.

• **Warning.** If taken in excess, vervain can cause vomiting. It is not recommended for use during pregnancy.

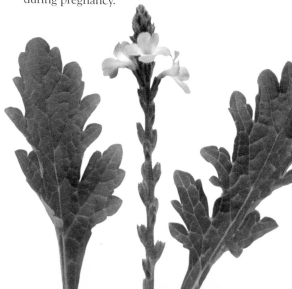

Headache fighting foods

Headaches are not isolated occurrences. They are symptoms
of a number of physical and mental imbalances.
One root cause can be your diet. Eating a balanced diet
is fundamental in preventing and fighting headaches.

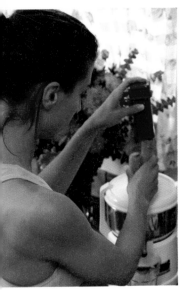

✚ Low blood sugar levels can cause
headaches. This is why maintaining a
balanced level of sugar in the blood is
important. This is not refined sugar but
carbohydrates and fructose sugars that
benefit the body (for example, from
fruit). Some people who suffer from
frequent headaches and migraines may
be sensitive to certain food chemicals,
both naturally occurring and artificial. If
you suffer from headaches try avoiding
foods that contain tiramines, common
compounds found in a wide range of
foods, including spinach, tomato,
potato, small whole fish, tuna, liver,
dark chocolate and alcoholic drinks, that
affect the arteries in the head. The most
common foods that have been found to bring
on headaches are alcohol (beer in particular),
chocolate, aged cheeses, brewer's yeast,
aged/cured meats, sausages and herrings.
Copper rich foods have also been found to
cause headaches, because they transport
tiramines through the body, causing pain.
Among those, **dried fruits**, **wheat germ**
and **shellfish** are included; similarly, **citrus
fruits** can also increase the body's absorption
of copper.

NOTE
You should always
consult your doctor
before changing
your diet.

Other factors that provoke headaches are working in low lighting. In this case try to eat plenty of carotene which is found in **carrots**, leucoanthocyanins found in **grapes** and bilberry anthocyanins which can fortify your sight and eye health.

An overworked liver from removing toxins may be the cause of headaches; which is why it is important to avoid excess alcohol, fried and fatty foods. There are foods that tend to bring on intense headaches, which is why eating a balanced diet rich in nutrients might help to prevent and fight headaches.

VITAMINS AND MINERALS

Vitamins are organic substances with carbon, necessary for the process of breaking down calories and providing nutrients for living organisms. They don't provide our bodies with energy because they do not contain any calories. They can't be used as fuel, but without vitamins and minerals our bodies couldn't absorb the cell constructing and energy compounds we get from food. This is why vitamins and minerals are considered nutrients.

When we don't ingest the necessary amount of vitamins and minerals in our daily diets, we may suffer from physical ailments as a result; headaches can be one of these. Headaches may be the result of a deficiency of the essential vitamins and minerals that we need for our physical and mental balance and health. This is why a deficiency can cause pain. Including extra vitamins and minerals may help in the treatment and prevention of headaches. We have put together a guide to fundamental nutrients that might help to fight headaches:

OATMEAL A POTENT CEREAL

Oatmeal is recommended for fighting headaches and nervous ailments. It is rich in vitamins B_1, B_2, E, PP and D, in addition to niacin, carotene, sulfur, calcium, phosphorus, potassium, sodium, iron, magnesium, copper and zinc. Because it is high in phosphorus, oatmeal is a very good food for supporting brain activity.

OATMEAL SOUP
(for 2 servings)
Add 2 or 3 tablespoons of oatmeal to a stock of carrots and squash. Allow to cook for 2 minutes and garnish with seaweed powder.

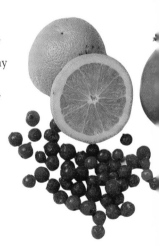

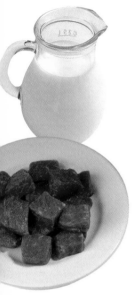

Vitamin B$_1$

This vitamin is fundamental for the function of the nervous system; a lack of this nutrient may cause headaches, nervousness, lack of concentration, exhaustion and different types of nervous disturbance. You can get the necessary daily amount of vitamin B$_1$ by including **oatmeal** or **wholewheat bread** into your daily diet. Every 3^1/$_2$ oz/100 g of oatmeal contains 0,40 mg of vitamin B$_1$ (the same amount of white bread contains 0.09mg). B$_1$ can be found in **meats, egg yolks, liver, milk, wholegrain cereals, sunflower seeds, beans, vegetables** and **yeast**.

Vitamin B$_2$

A deficiency of this vitamin can provoke eye strain and headaches. As with all B complex vitamins, it has a relaxing effect and fights insomnia and headaches caused by postural tension, it is also an important vitamin for the skin. It is found in **spinach** (not frozen), **broccoli, dairy products, meats, fish, eggs, brown rice, soy flour, alfalfa sprouts, green vegetables** and **kidney beans**.

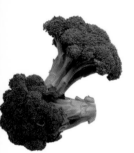

HEALTHY BREAKFAST

Dissolve ^{1}/$_2$ teaspoon of yeast in 1 cup of tepid water and add 2 tablespoons of oil (preferably olive oil) and sea salt. Add this mixture to 4 cups of wholewheat flour and mix until you have a stiff dough, so that it doesn't stick to the bowl. Add the amount of warm water necessary (approximately 2 cups of water). Let the dough rise for ^{1}/$_2$ hour and knead it again. Form small rolls with your hands, place on a rectangular baking sheet and let sit for another 30 minutes. Bake at a moderate temperature.

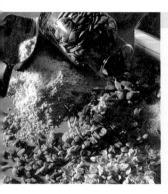

WHOLE GRAINS

Thus called because they are unprocessed grains, that is, the wheat grain, or the seeds and shells are not removed. They are helpful in preventing and fighting headaches, because, thanks to the fibers, they help to maintain a balanced level of blood sugar in the body. To prevent headaches, it is important to incorporate into your breakfast oatmeal, rye, wholegrain cereals, etc. In addition, whole grains help to fight mental fatigue and are rich in vitamins B and E and the minerals calcium, iron and zinc.

Vitamin B₃

Studies have shown that this vitamin helps to prevent and relieve headaches. This vitamin is fundamental for supporting the blood vessels' function. Deficiency produces symptoms of nervousness and stress. Niacin (or vitamin B_3) is not destroyed by heat, light, air or basic solutions. However, it's easily flushed out of the body by water, making it a water-soluble vitamin. It is found in **fish, beans, wholewheat flour, soy, oatmeal, corn, tomatoes, potatoes, alfalfa** and **meats**.

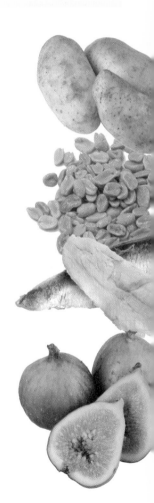

Vitamin B₅

This acid belongs to the B complex vitamin group, water-soluble vitamins with different functions. It helps to develop the nervous system, to release energy from foods and to convert fats and sugars into energy. Deficiency provokes hypoglycemia, and as a result, headaches. It also helps to prevent fatigue. Recommended daily dose is 6 mg, although athletes should get more vitamin B_5, because they use more energy. Vitamin B_5 rich foods include **meats**, especially **liver, poultry, fish; fresh fruit, dairy products, cereals** and **vegetables**.

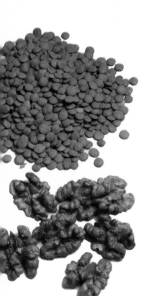

Vitamin B₆

This vitamin is necessary for increasing the levels of serotonin (natural chemical found in the brain) that acts as an anti-depressant and as a neurotransmitter, lowering the risk of continuous pain. Various studies have shown that B_6 can be used to fight headaches and mental fatigue. If taken in capsules, you shouldn't exceed 200 mg per day. It is found in **potatoes**, **bananas**, **wholegrain cereals**, **raisins**, **lentils**, **peanuts**, **liver**, **turkey** and **tuna**.

Vitamin B₁₂

Deficiency symptoms can take 2 to 3 years to develop and are clinically recognized for their effect on the nervous system, causing irritability, which can bring on tension headaches. Also called cyanocobamin, it is an important vitamin in the forming of red blood cells and the regeneration of tissue. Because it is hydro-soluble, up to 30 percent of vitamin B_{12} is lost when meat and fish are boiled. Basic food sources include **liver**, **meats**, **fish**, **entrails**, **eggs** and

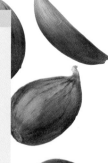

GARLIC

Allicin is the most powerful active component found in garlic; it also contains enzymes and aminoacids, which have prolonged antibacterial action. It is also abundant in minerals such as zinc and magnesium and vitamins C, A, B_1, B_2, PP and E. It stimulates the production of bile (which helps to calm stomach cramps) and improves your appetite. Garlic supports digestion, fights against swelling, gas, stimulates gastric secretions and strengthens the stomach and intestinal lining. It's important to know that for garlic to have potent effects, it's best to use garlic over time, eating 3 cloves of garlic a day, 900 mg of garlic powder or 9 capsules.

in small quantities, **milk** and other **dairy products**; distributing these foods in a balanced way can cover the body's needs for this vitamin.

Vitamin C

The amount of vitamin C in the body decreases when under stress; this is why a proper intake of vitamin C is important for people who are under a lot of stress, to prevent colds and headaches. It is calculated that eating one citrus fruit a day is enough (but not before meals because it increases the absorption of copper by the body, which generates headaches). Vitamin C should be consumed daily since it doesn't accumulate. It is found in **citrus fruits**, some **vegetables**, **strawberries**, **kiwis**, **guavas**, **currants**, **oranges**, **tomatoes** and **red peppers**.

Vitamin E

Also called "alpha tocopherol", this vitamin is fat-soluble and is essential for the body, it helps to prevent headaches caused by eye strain. In general, it maintains the body's health by protecting the body from toxic molecules resulting from normal metabolism, ones that enter the body through the respiratory system and mouth. It is mostly found in **egg yolks**, **vegetable oils** (**soy**, **peanut**, **rice**, **cotton** and **coconut**), **celery**, **green leafy vegetables**, **cereals** (especially **wheat germ**) and **wholegrain breads**.

BENEFICIAL LIVER

Liver is the most important source of vitamin B_{12}. Although it tends not to be included in the daily diet, there are ways to prepare liver as a tasty treat.

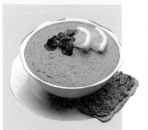

PATÉ EXPRESS
Sauté a liver, and then grind it or use a hand held blender, add 1/2 shredded or finely chopped onion add 1 chopped hardboiled egg, add salt and pepper to taste. This is a very tasty paté to put on toasted wholewheat bread.

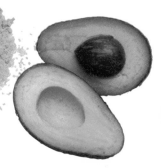

Folic acid

This vitamin belongs to the B group and is water-soluble. It can't be produced or stored inside the body, which is why it needs to be included in the daily diet. A lack of this vitamin can affect the nervous system (producing permanent nervousness, insomnia and headaches caused by tension). It is beneficial during menopause, intervening by increasing levels of estrogen, which may cause headaches and overall exhaustion. It is a fundamental vitamin during pregnancy and breastfeeding. It might provide benefits in the treatment of liver diseases, tumors, alcoholism and lack of vitamin C and B_{12}. It is found in **green leafy vegetables**, **garden vegetables**, **fruits**, **beans**, and **potatoes** (since this vitamin is destroyed by heat, it's best to eat fresh foods, without cooking or with only minimal cooking).

MIRACULOUS CELERY

Celery is great vegetable that might relieve your headaches and other ailments caused by stressful situations. Its composition is rich in potassium, phosphorus and vitamins C, B₁ and E, which makes it a great food against intense headaches, because these active components can calm pain. In medieval times it was considered a miracle plant, because of its ability to clear the mind and fortify the spirit. Today it is proven that the tranquilizing properties of its essential nutrients can help to regulate the functions of the central nervous system. Because of its diuretic qualities, it contributes to fighting headaches caused by high blood pressure. **Warning.** It is not recommended to expose your skin to direct sunlight after eating a lot of celery, because it makes your skin more sensitive to the sun.

CALMING JUICE

Boil a celery plant for 2 minutes. Cut it in pieces and place it in a juicer to extract the juice (which you should drink 2 times a day). You can also blend a fresh plant in a blender (roots, stalks and leaves), with enough water. Drink 2 or 3 times a day. This juice can help to calm headaches.

Zinc

Component of insulin, which is consumed faster when you are in stressful situations. Deficiency can cause headaches. It is found in **garlic, oysters, aloe vera, pumpkinseeds, ginger, lamb, liver, green peas, milk, egg yolks** and **parsley**.

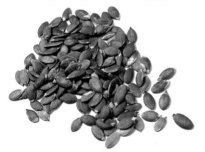
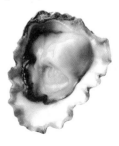

Chrome

When the body lacks this mineral it is very possible that insulin levels in the body will become disrupted and that the breakdown of carbohydrates, aminoacids and fats will change. Chrome works along side insulin to regulate blood sugar levels; it decreases the amount of fat and increases muscular mass. It is found in **egg yolks, red meat, wheat, wholewheat flour** and **molasses**.

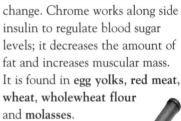

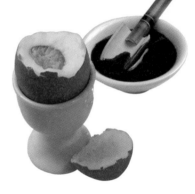

CIDER VINEGAR

Vinegar, in all its varieties, has been used for hundreds of years not only as a condiment but also as a drink and natural remedy. It contains minerals and microelements such as calcium, phosphorus, magnesium, sodium, and silicon; it is rich in potassium. It has regenerative and curative properties which are the result of the synergy of all its active ingredients. It is used for chronic headaches.

AGAINST MIGRAINES
Add 2 tablespoons of cider vinegar and 1 spoonful of honey to 1 glass of hot water and mix. Drink 2 or 3 glasses of this mixture a day, in small sips, to calm chronic headaches.

Phosphorus

This mineral is the most abundant in the body, after calcium. It is fundamental for the body's chemical reactions because it captures, transfers and stores energy. It is very important for nerve tissue, supporting the nervous system's functions and helping to recover from mental fatigue accompanied by headaches and from difficult concentrating. Deficiency causes memory loss, dizziness and migraines. For it to be properly absorbed

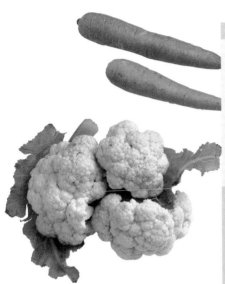

into the body it's best to combine it with calcium and vitamin D. Phosphorus rich foods include **cod fish**, **milk**, **dairy products**, **wholegrain cereals**, **nuts**, **almonds**, **peanuts**, **figs**, **mushrooms**, **celery**, **onion**, **cauliflower**, **parsley** and **leeks**.

Iron

Lack of iron causes physical and mental fatigue, headaches and irritability. One of its main functions is to take oxygen to the tissues and brain, which is why a lack of iron can cause pain and nervous tension. It intervenes in the action of breathing; it combines with proteins to form red blood cells and to transport oxygen. It is recommended that those who suffer from headaches and tension ingest iron because it activates vitamins from the B group and stimulates physical resistance. It is found in **seaweed**, **liver**, **eggs**, **spinach**, **lentils** and **sardines**.

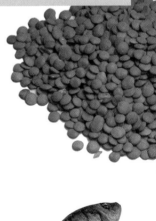

Magnesium

An important anti-stress nutrient, which helps to keep the blood veins healthy. It reduces the nerves' excitability and promotes muscle relaxation. It helps to prevent headaches associated with tension and nervousness. It also helps to fight against irritability. Magnesium deficiency tends to be associated with other nutrient deficiencies, caused by a poor diet full of frozen and processed foods. It is found in **brown sugar, almonds, whole cereals, nuts, soy beans, sesame seeds, dried figs** and **green garden vegetables**.

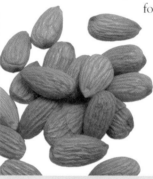

PEAR MOUSE
Dissolve 2 tablespoons of rice flour in 1 glass of milk and place over the stove in a pot, while you add 1 teaspoon of sugar. When it comes to a boil, take it off the stove and add a grated or blended pear, lemon rind from $1/2$ lemon and 1 egg white whipped until firm. Mix gently with a wooden spatula. Distribute to cups and if you wish refrigerate. This mouse can be served room temperature or chilled.

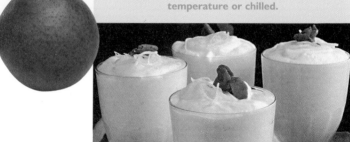

Potassium

Essential mineral for the nervous system. Deficiency can cause headaches, provoked by nervousness and chronic stress. It can also produce insomnia and depression. It is found in **celery**, **cauliflower**, **lettuce**, **beans**, **bananas**, **dates** and **spinach**.

SUNFLOWER SEEDS

Seeds from this flower are rich in vitamin E, phosphorus, magnesium and potassium, they can be very good for fighting headaches and dizziness. They are aromatic and tasty; they can be eaten raw or roasted and salted. They can also be added to various baked goods.

Warning. They are high in fats, which gives them lubricating and laxative properties. As a result, people with digestive problems should eat them in moderation.

SWEET PAIN RELIEVER
Roughly grind $^1/_2$ tablespoon of sunflower seeds, and mix them with 1 tablespoon sugar. Add water and drink before going to bed.

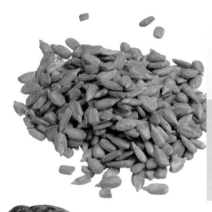

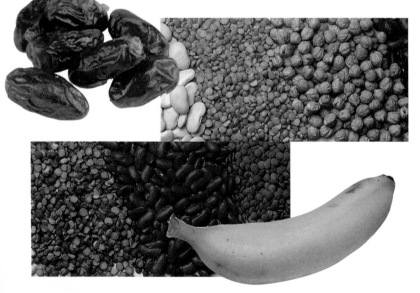

Detoxifying diet

A weekly detoxifying diet can be a great way to accompany a treatment for headaches, because it cleans toxins from the body and energizes the mind and body. This diet is indicated only if the person is healthy and has consulted his doctor.

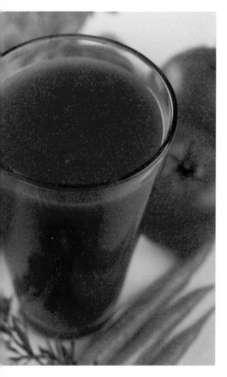

This is a basic diet, rich in vegetables and lean proteins. The dishes are based on salads and grains such as soy, wheat and brown rice. For breakfast and snacks, fruit juices and vegetables.

Basic rules

- For breakfast drink natural orange or carrot juice with $1/2$ cup of each one (see recipe on page 59).
- For snacks, alternate different juices (for example, lemon, grapefruit, apple and orange). Each day drink a different fruit juice.
- For lunch and dinner, eat varied salads, trying to mix them up each day. They can be accompanied by soy burgers (or other soy, wheat or rice based dishes), walnuts and 3 eggs a week.
- A healthy dressing for salads includes olive or raw sunflower oil, lemon, vinegar and salt.
- For desert: gelatin or mint tea.

CARROTS AND ORANGES

Prepare breakfast juice with $1/2$ cup of orange juice and $1/2$ cup of carrot juice (which can be extracted from 2 small carrots, peeled and chopped). If you use a juicer, you shouldn't add any water. If you are using a blender, add a little bit of water for texture. Add to this juice 1 tablespoon of wheat germ, mixed very well. **Drink before eating breakfast.**

LIGHT DINNERS

Garden salads are rich in basic vegetables and are a great detoxifying food. They are a great option for a light dinner and can be combined with other dishes. It's best to choose veggies that are in season, because they are fresher, delicious and more economical.

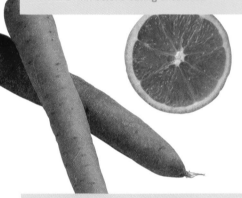

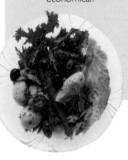

MONDAY

BREAKFAST
- A natural orange and carrot juice (see recipe).

LUNCH
Garden salad
- Boil a small white cabbage for 3 minutes. Separately, boil a 1 lb/500 g package of frozen peas. And also separately 4 green zucchinis (after cooking soak in cold water to stop the cooking process). Cut the zucchini in cubes and place all the ingredients in a salad bowl, with 2 small carrots thinly sliced (almost transparent), 2 chopped tomatoes, a small amount of celery in small slices and a bunch of green leafy lettuce. Dress with a vinaigrette prepared with olive oil, cider vinegar, salt and pepper.

SNACK
- Apple juice.

DINNER
Soy patties with tomato and basil salad
- Slice several ripe tomatoes (but fresh) and add a spoonfull of olive oil, 1 of vinegar, salt and black pepper. Sprinkle with basil leaves cut up with your hands.

TUESDAY

BREAKFAST
* A natural orange and carrot juice (see recipe on page 59).

LUNCH
Roasted pepper salad
* Roast several red and green peppers ahead of time (you can use several cooking methods: in the oven, on the stove, covered with aluminum foil, in a frying pan, on the grill or in the microwave; the secret is to burn the skin, so that you can remove it easily). When they are roasted, peeled and cooled down, cut them into long strips and add cherry tomatoes, finely chopped onion and crushed garlic. Dress with salt and olive oil.

SNACK
* Grapefruit juice.

DINNER
Soy burgers with tabbouleh (a Middle Eastern salad with wheat and herbs)
* Soak for an hour 6 oz/180 g of bulgur wheat in cold water, drain and press with your hands. Separately, chop 8 spring onions without the green parts, 3 tomatoes and 1 large sprig of fresh parsley, without the stems. Mix with the bulgur wheat and dress with a vinaigrette prepared with olive oil, lemon juice, salt and black pepper. This tabbouleh can accompany soy burgers (see recipe).

RICE BALLS

Beyond being nutritious and filling, brown rice can also be used to make balls. Mix cooked rice with I onion marinated in oil and dress with salt, pepper and chopped parsley. Mix the ingredients well and prepare balls with your hands. Brown the balls in a pan or in the oven, on both sides.

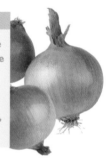

SOY BURGERS
Mash 2 cups of cooked soy beans, still hot and mix with 2 cups of cooked brown rice (also still hot), garlic and fresh chopped parsley. Add a pinch of sea salt and I teaspoon of oregano to taste. With your hands form hamburger patties and bread with breadcrumbs. Bake in the oven at a high temperature for approximately I0 minutes.

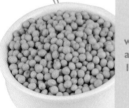

WEDNESDAY

BREAKFAST
- A natural orange and carrot juice (see recipe on page 59).

LUNCH
Tao salad
- Cut in very fine strips 8 leaves of Chinese cabbage, 1 turnip, 2 celery stalks, 2 carrots (they should be very tender), 2 round zucchinis and a small piece of ginger. Boil 7 oz/200 g of white rice for 5 minutes and drain. Place all of the ingredients in a steamer and when the rice is almost ready, add 3 1/2 oz/100 g of bean sprouts and allow to sit for a few minutes. Remove from the steamer and allow to cool down. Dress with sesame   or soy oil and soy sauce.

SNACK
- Lemon juice.

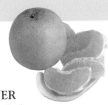

DINNER
Wholegrain rice balls with mushroom salad
- Wash well 7 oz/200 g of mushrooms and slice. Dress with a marinade of olive oil, lemon juice, 1 teaspoon of chopped onion, chopped parsley, chopped tarragon, salt and pepper. Accompany with rice balls (see recipe on page 60).

THURSDAY

BREAKFAST
- A natural orange and carrot juice (see recipe on page 59).

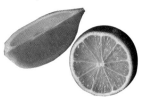

LUNCH
Bean salad
- Soak over night and cook with plenty of water and a touch of salt each separately 8 oz/250 g chick peas, 8 oz/250 g lentils and 8 oz/250 g of white beans. When they are tender, drain and cool down. Make a salad with 1 onion and 2 carrots sliced julian style. Dress with olive oil, vinegar and salt.

SNACK
- Orange juice.

DINNER
Light salad
- Wash well and tear up with your hands a bunch of butterhead lettuce, endives, spinach, watercress, arugula, celery, cherry tomatoes, heart of palm and white asparagus. Dress with olive oil and fresh herbs.

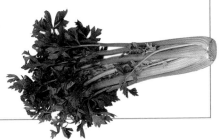

FRIDAY

BREAKFAST
- A natural orange and carrot juice (see recipe on page 59).

LUNCH
Light salad
- Cook separately 3¹/₂ oz/100 g of potatoes, 3¹/₂ oz/100 g of peas, 3¹/₂ oz/100 g white beans add 3¹/₂ oz/100 g and 3¹/₂ oz/100 g sweet peas. Once cooked and cooled down, mix in a salad with diced tomatoes and 1 sliced small onion in rings; dress with olive oil, salt and vinegar.

SNACK
- Apple juice.

DINNER
Green tart and squash salad
- For the tart, prepare a dough with soy (see recipe on page 63) and fill with your favorite vegetables.
- For a salad cut a squash in half and brown in the oven with olive oil, salt and pepper. Take out of the oven and set to cool. Serve with radish leaves and soaked sun dried tomatoes.

SATURDAY

BREAKFAST
- A natural orange and carrot juice (see recipe on page 59).

LUNCH
Braised salad
- Roast in the oven or grill 1 whole onion, 1 pepper, 1 zucchini and 1 eggplant. Allow to cool, remove the skin and cut in strips. Add chopped garlic, salt and olive oil.

SNACK
- Grapefruit juice.

DINNER
Soy patties with cheese and sweet salad
- For the salad, peel and cut into slices 3 apples and 2 carrots. Dress with olive oil, salt, lemon and a few drops of soy sauce. Another delicious combination is oranges and onions, dressed with the same dressing. (See recipe for soy patties).

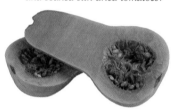

EASY SOY PATTIES

Prepare a mixture with 8 oz/250 g of cooked and mashed soy beans, 10 oz/300 g of wholewheat flour, sea salt, garlic, parsley and oregano. Use a rolling pin to make a thin dough. Use a large cup or cut patties with a knife and boil for a few minutes (until they float). Remove from the water and bread with breadcrumbs. You can cook the patties in a pan or in the oven, alone or covered with tomato sauce.

WHEAT AND TOFU BURGERS

Mix 2 cups of bulgur wheat cooked, with a block of firm tofu, I clove of garlic and I grated onion. Add salt, chopped parsley and other spices such as cumin or curry. Make a dough and form hamburgers. Bake in the oven.

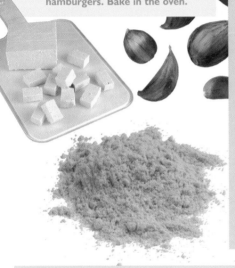

SOY DOUGH FOR TARTS

Mix in a bowl 8 oz/250 g of wholewheat flour and 3 tablespoons of soy flour with I pinch of sea salt. Separately dissolve I tablespoon of yeast in I cup of tepid water and add 2 tablespoons of oil. Add to the flour and form a dough, adding the amount of tepid water necessary. Allow the dough to sit and rise for 1/2 hour; roll the dough with a rolling pin; and place the dough in a greased tart pan and fill with your favorite vegetables (you can use this same mixture to make filled pastries).

SUNDAY

BREAKFAST
• A natural orange and carrot juice (see recipe on page 59).

LUNCH
Multicolor salad
• Wash a package of asparagus, cut off the end of the stems and cook in boiling water for 15 minutes. Separately, boil 4 corn cobs and 3 eggs. Place in a salad bowl one green curled lettuce, thinly sliced and 2 green apples, diced. Add the corn cut from the cob, chopped hardboiled eggs and the asparagus. Dress with olive oil, salt and pepper.

SNACK
• Orange juice.

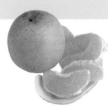

DINNER
Wheat and tofu burgers with spinach salad
• Wash 7oz/200 g of spinach; thinly sliced and add to a salad bowl, along with a few sun dried tomatoes and pine nuts previously browned in a pan. Dress with a dressing made with 1 chopped clove of garlic, olive oil, lemon juice, salt and pepper.

index

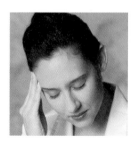